Elimination diet cookbook for seniors over 40-60

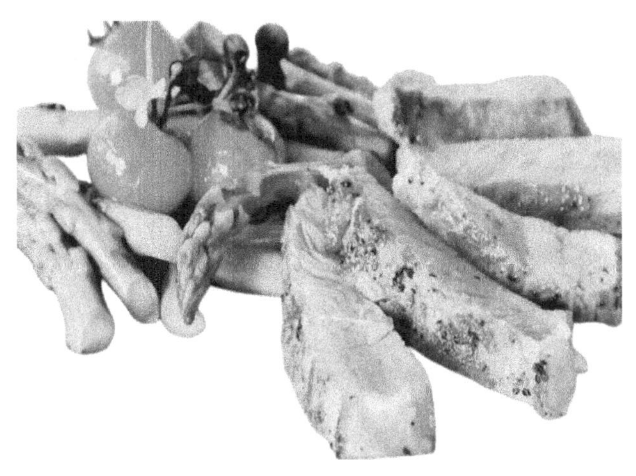

Identify those foods that make sicky all time, to have a healthy lifestyle that is Fatigue free, poor brain function and more . With over 150 recipes and 4 weeks of food, eliminate meal plans just for you.

Dr.Raymond Harris

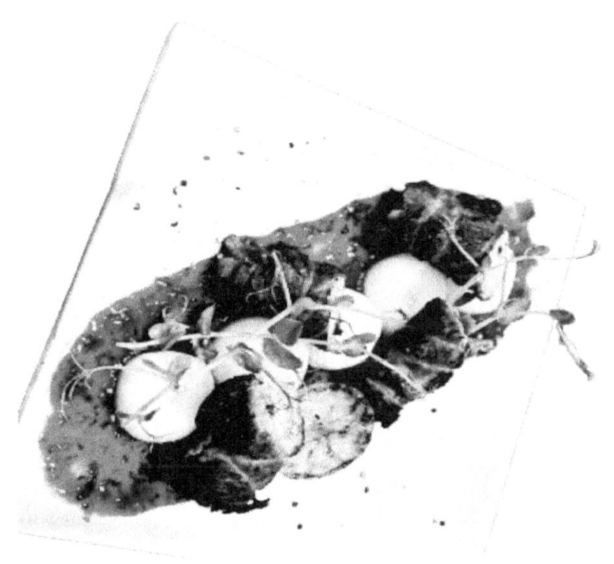

Table of content

Introduction to Elimination Diets for Seniors

As people become older, the significance of consuming a diet that is both nutritious and balanced becomes more important.
When it comes to diet, senior citizens, who are typically between the ages of 40 and 60, often have particular health concerns that call for a deliberate approach.
 The elimination diet is one such dietary regimen that is becoming more popular among middle-aged and elderly people.

In this extensive introduction, we will dig into the advantages and concerns that are special to senior citizens who are beginning an elimination diet. Our goal is to shed light on how this strategy may help to the general well-being of senior citizens.

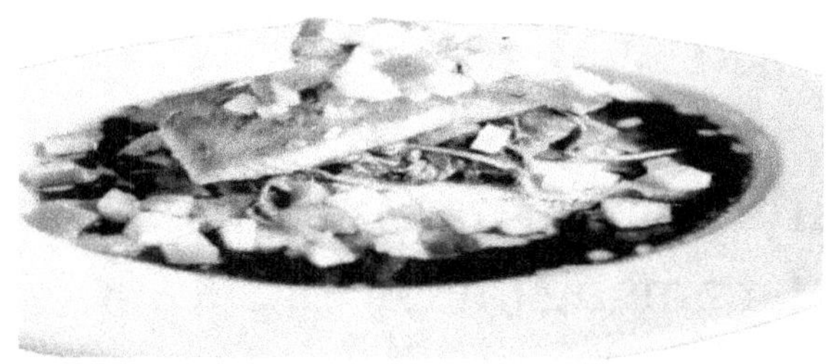

chapter one

What You Need to Know About the Elimination Diet

This is a planned eating plan that is aimed to identify and remove possible trigger foods that may be producing unfavorable responses in the body. The elimination diet is also known as the elimination diet. Some of the symptoms that may be caused by these responses include digestive problems, inflammation, joint discomfort, and other symptoms that have an effect on general health.

In order to examine individual reactions, the technique entails deliberately eliminating certain food categories or specific substances from the diet for a predetermined amount of time, and then gradually reintroducing these products throughout the subsequent period.

Adaptation for Senior Citizens

1. Nutrient Density for Aging Bodies

Seniors typically experience issues relating to nutrition intake and preserving muscular mass. An elimination diet suited for this age group emphasizes nutrient-dense foods, ensuring kids acquire appropriate vitamins and minerals needed for bone development, immunological function, and general vigor.

2. Digestive Sensitivity in Aging

The digestive tract undergoes changes with age, and seniors may have heightened sensitivity to particular meals. An elimination diet helps individuals to detect and eliminate triggers, enhancing digestive comfort and nutritional absorption.

3. Addressing Age-Related
Inflammation

Inflammation is a significant problem
as persons age, leading to many health
complications. The elimination diet
may serve as a strong tool for seniors to
identify and remove inflammatory
foods, possibly easing joint discomfort
and lowering the risk of chronic
illnesses connected with inflammation.

Benefits of Elimination Diets for Seniors

1. Customized Approach to Health

The customized nature of elimination diets allows seniors to adjust their eating patterns to their unique health demands. This personalization may lead to greater energy levels, better digestion, and enhanced general well-being.

2. Identification of Food Sensitivities

Seniors may acquire allergies to specific foods over time. The elimination diet offers a methodical technique to identify and remove possible triggers, helping elders manage and reduce symptoms connected to food sensitivities.

3. Weight Management and
Metabolism Support

  As metabolism tends to slow down
with age, weight control becomes a
problem for many seniors. The
elimination diet, when done with a
focus on balanced nutrition, may help
healthy weight control by boosting the
intake of nutrient-dense foods and
eliminating possible inflammatory
factors.

4. Enhanced Cognitive Function

  Certain foods have been related to
cognitive decline, and seniors might

benefit from identifying and removing these possible factors via an exclusion diet. Emphasizing brain-boosting nutrients may further promote cognitive wellness.

Considerations for Seniors

1. Medical Supervision

Before beginning on any substantial dietary changes, seniors should speak with healthcare specialists, particularly if they have pre-existing health concerns or are taking medicines that may be influenced by dietary alterations.

2. Balancing Nutrient Intake

Ensuring elders acquire appropriate nutrition is vital. The elimination diet should be carefully prepared to avoid nutritional deficits, considering the special dietary demands of this age group.

3. Gradual Introduction of Foods

Reintroducing removed foods should be a progressive process, enabling seniors to evaluate how their bodies respond to each reintroduction.

This careful method helps pinpoint particular triggers without overloading the system.

Ten suggestions for a healthy you

1. Prioritize Nutrient-Rich Foods:
   Focus on a balanced diet rich in fruits, vegetables, whole grains, lean meats, and healthy fats. Nutrient-dense meals supply important vitamins and minerals for general well-being.

2. Stay Hydrated: Maintain optimal hydration by consuming a sufficient quantity of water throughout the day. Water is necessary for several body

activities, including digestion, circulation, and temperature control.

3. Regular Physical Activity: Incorporate regular exercise into your regimen, aiming for a balance of aerobic, strength, and flexibility training. Physical exercise leads to enhanced mood, greater energy, and general wellness.

4. Adequate Sleep: Prioritize quality sleep by adopting a regular sleep routine and creating a sleep-friendly atmosphere. Sufficient rest is vital for bodily and mental regeneration.

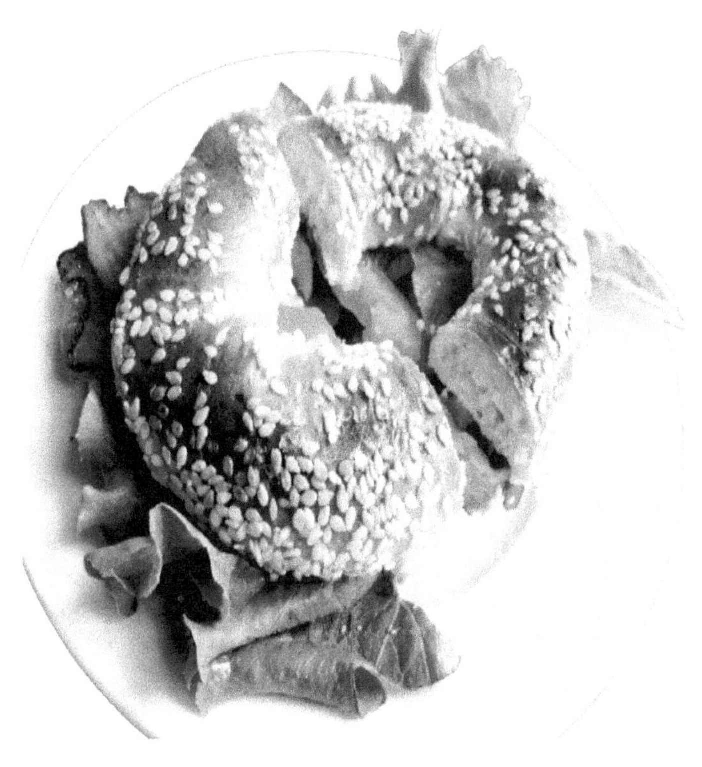

5. Mindful Eating: Practice mindful eating by paying attention to hunger and fullness indicators. Avoid distractions when eating, appreciate each mouthful, and be careful of portion sizes to build a better connection with food.

6. Stress Management: Develop effective stress management strategies, such as deep breathing, meditation, or yoga. Chronic stress may significantly effect both physical and mental health, so finding healthy strategies to cope is crucial.

7. Social ties: Cultivate meaningful
relationships and social ties. Positive
social connections contribute to mental
well-being and may even have physical
health advantages.

8. Regular Health Check-ups:
 Schedule frequent health check-ups
and tests to monitor your well-being
and spot any health concerns early.
Prevention and early intervention are
crucial to preserving healthy health.

9. Limit Processed meals and Added
Sugars: Reduce your consumption of
processed meals and foods rich in
added sugars. Opt for complete,
unprocessed meals to offer your body

with important nutrients without unneeded additions.

10. Continuous Learning and Mental Stimulation: Keep your mind active and engaged by seeking continuous learning, whether by reading, taking up a new hobby, or engaging in activities that test your cognitive talents. Mental stimulation is vital for brain health as you age.

Chapter two

Some meals to consume

1. Leafy Greens: Incorporate spinach, kale, collard greens, and other leafy greens rich in vitamins, minerals, and antioxidants for general health.

2. Berries: Enjoy a range of berries such as blueberries, strawberries, and raspberries. They are filled with antioxidants and help to heart health.

3. Oily Fish: Include fatty fish like salmon, mackerel, and sardines in

your diet for omega-3 fatty acids, which promote heart and brain function.

4. Nuts and Seeds: Snack on almonds, walnuts, chia seeds, and flaxseeds. These contain healthful fats, fiber, and important nutrients.

5. Whole Grains: Choose whole grains like quinoa, brown rice, oats, and whole wheat for sustained energy and an excellent source of fiber.

6. Colorful Vegetables: Consume a variety of colorful vegetables, such as bell peppers, carrots, and sweet potatoes, to provide a varied range of nutrients.

7. Lean Proteins: Opt for lean protein sources like chicken, tofu, beans, and lentils to promote muscular health and keep you feeling full.

8. Greek Yogurt: Include Greek yogurt for a protein-rich dairy choice that also delivers probiotics for digestive health.

9. Avocado: Add avocado to your meals for healthy monounsaturated fats, contributing to heart health and satiety.

10. Tomatoes: Incorporate tomatoes, which are high in antioxidants like lycopene, into salads, sauces, or snacks for possible cancer-fighting effects.

Some meals you shouldn't consume

1. Highly Processed Foods: Limit consumption of excessively processed foods rich in additives, preservatives, and artificial components, since they typically lack vital nutrients and may lead to health difficulties.

2. Added Sugars: Reduce consumption of foods and drinks with high added sugar content, since excessive sugar intake is connected to several health risks, including obesity and diabetes.

3. Trans Fats: Avoid trans fats
contained in partly hydrogenated oils,
often present in many fried and
commercially baked goods. Trans fats
may elevate harmful cholesterol levels
and increase the risk of heart disease.

4. Sugary Beverages: Minimize the use
of sugary beverages such sodas and
fruit juices, since they may lead to
weight gain and have detrimental
effects on metabolic health.

5. Processed Meats: Limit the
consumption of processed meats such
as sausages,

bacon, and hot dogs, since they typically include additives and may be connected to an increased risk of certain health conditions, including cancer.

6. Excessive Red Meat: While red meat may be part of a balanced diet, eating it excessively may be connected with an elevated risk of certain health issues. Opt for lean cuts and seek plant-based protein sources.

7. Highly Salted meals: Cut down on meals with high sodium content, since excessive salt consumption is related to high blood pressure and may lead to cardiovascular difficulties.

8. Artificial Sweeteners:
  Be careful with artificial sweeteners contained in certain diet products, since their long-term effects are still under research, and they may impair metabolism and gut health for some people.

9. Highly Refined Grains: Choose whole grains over refined grains like white flour, since they retain more nutrients and fiber. Highly processed carbohydrates may contribute to fast rises in blood sugar.

10. Fast Food and Fried goods: Limit fast food and fried goods, which generally include harmful fats, excessive calories, and may lead to weight gain and other health concerns when eaten consistently.

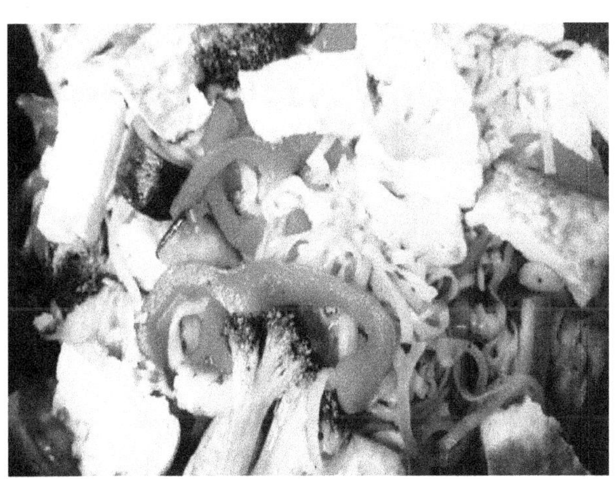

Chapter three

Senior friendly recipes

1. Easy Vegetable Stir-Fry:
1. ngredients: Mixed veggies (broccoli, carrots, bell peppers), tofu or chicken, low-sodium soy sauce, garlic, ginger.

  Quick to make and full with bright vegetables, this stir-fry is both healthful and easy on the teeth.

2. Quinoa Salad with Avocado and Chickpeas:

  Ingredients: Quinoa, chickpeas, cucumber, cherry tomatoes, avocado, olive oil, lemon juice.

A light and protein-packed salad delivering a range of textures and tastes.

3. Baked Salmon with Lemon and Dill:
   Ingredients: Salmon fillets, lemon, fresh dill, olive oil, garlic.
   Simple and heart-healthy, this baked salmon dish is rich in omega-3 fatty acids.

4 10. Sweet Potato and Kale Hash:
Ingredients: Sweet potatoes, kale, onions, garlic, olive oil, paprika.
   Instructions: Sauté sweet potatoes, kale, and onions with garlic and paprika for a tasty and healthy hash.

Meat recipes

1. Grilled Lemon Herb Chicken:
Ingredients: Chicken breasts, lemon,
garlic, rosemary, thyme, olive oil.

Instructions: Marinate chicken with
lemon, garlic, and herbs; grill to
perfection for a juicy and tasty main
dish.

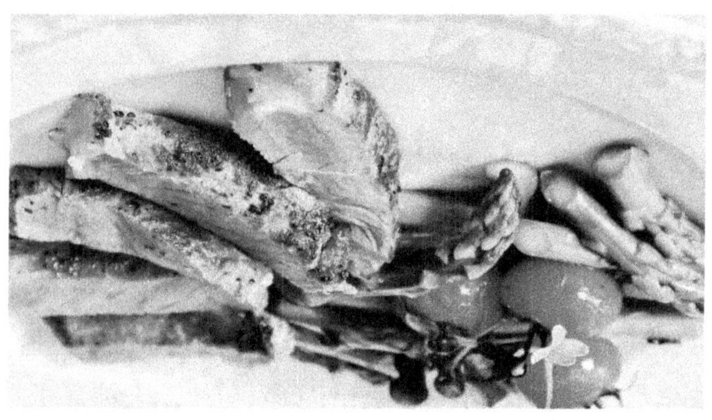

2. Beef and Broccoli Stir-Fry:
   Ingredients: Beef strips, broccoli,
soy sauce, ginger, garlic, sesame oil.
   Instructions: Stir-fry beef and
broccoli in a flavorful blend of soy
sauce, ginger, and garlic for a fast and
tasty supper.

3. Baked Honey Mustard Salmon:
Ingredients: Salmon fillets, honey,
Dijon mustard, lemon, herbs.
   Instructions: Mix honey, mustard,
lemon, and herbs; coat fish and bake
for a sweet and tangy seafood meal.

4. pasta Bolognese: Ingredients: Ground meat, tomatoes, onions, garlic, Italian herbs, whole wheat pasta.

Instructions: Cook beef with tomatoes, onions, and herbs; serve over whole wheat spaghetti for a traditional and hearty pasta meal.

5. Herb-Crusted Pork Chops: Ingredients: Pork chops, breadcrumbs, thyme, rosemary, garlic, olive oil.

Instructions: Coat pork chops with a herb-infused breadcrumb mixture;

bake or grill until golden brown for a tasty main meal.

6. Turkey and Vegetable Skewers:
Ingredients: Ground turkey, bell peppers, red onion, cherry tomatoes, olive oil, herbs.

Instructions: Mix turkey with seasonings; form into skewers with vegetables and cook for a lean and flavorful meal alternative.

7. Lemon Garlic Butter Shrimp Pasta:
Ingredients: Shrimp, whole wheat pasta, lemon, garlic, butter, cherry tomatoes.

Instructions: Sauté shrimp with garlic and lemon butter; serve with whole wheat pasta and cherry tomatoes for a wonderful seafood spaghetti.

8. Chicken and Vegetable Curry:
Ingredients: Chicken thighs, curry spices, coconut milk, bell peppers, carrots, onions.

Instructions: Cook chicken with curry spices, coconut milk, and veggies for a thick and fragrant curry.

9. Honey Dijon Glazed Chicken Thighs:
Ingredients: Chicken thighs, honey, Dijon mustard, garlic, herbs.

Instructions: Mix honey, Dijon, garlic, and herbs; cover chicken thighs and bake for a sweet and flavorful main meal.

10. Lamb Kebabs with Mint Yogurt Sauce:

Ingredients: Lamb cubes, yogurt, mint, garlic, cumin, coriander.

Instructions: Marinate lamb in yogurt, mint, garlic, cumin, and coriander; grill for a delicious and tender kebab.

Chapter four

Soup and stew recipes

1. Chicken and Vegetable Soup: Ingredients: Chicken broth, chicken breast, carrots, celery, onions, garlic, thyme.

Instructions: Simmer chicken and veggies in broth with thyme for a warm and healthful soup.

2. Beef and Barley Stew: Ingredients: Beef stew meat, barley, carrots, potatoes, onions, beef broth.

Instructions: Slow-cook meat, barley, and veggies in beef broth for a substantial and nourishing stew.

3. Tomato Basil Soup: Ingredients: Tomatoes, onions, garlic, vegetable broth, basil, cream.
   Instructions: Blend tomatoes, onions, and garlic; cook with broth, basil, and cream for a rich and aromatic tomato basil soup.

4. Lentil and Vegetable Stew: Ingredients: Lentils, carrots, tomatoes, celery, onions, vegetable broth, cumin.

Instructions: Cook lentils and veggies in broth with cumin for a protein-packed and hearty lentil stew.

5. Butternut Squash and Apple Soup:
Ingredients: Butternut squash, apples, onions, vegetable broth, nutmeg, cinnamon.
Instructions: Roast squash, apples, and onions; mix with broth, nutmeg, and cinnamon for a sweet and flavorful soup.

6. Minestrone Soup: Ingredients: Cannellini beans, tomatoes, zucchini, carrots, pasta, vegetable broth.

Instructions: Combine beans, veggies, pasta, and stock for a traditional and healthful minestrone soup.

7. Chicken and Rice Congee:
Ingredients: Chicken thighs, rice, ginger, garlic, chicken broth, green onions.
   Instructions: Simmer chicken, rice, and aromatics in broth; top with green onions for a soothing congee.

8. Spicy Black Bean Soup: Ingredients: Black beans, tomatoes, onions, garlic, chili powder, vegetable broth.
   Instructions: Cook black beans, tomatoes, and spices in broth for a spicy and tasty black bean soup.

9. Potato Leek Soup: Ingredients: Potatoes, leeks, onions, garlic, vegetable stock, thyme.

Instructions: Sauté leeks, onions, and garlic; simmer with potatoes, thyme, and broth for a creamy potato leek soup.

10. Moroccan Chickpea Stew: Ingredients: Chickpeas, tomatoes, carrots, bell peppers, onions, vegetable stock, Moroccan spices.

Instructions: Cook chickpeas and veggies in broth with Moroccan spices for a fragrant and hearty chickpea stew.

Snacks recipes

1. Greek Yogurt Parfait:
   Ingredients: Greek yogurt, granola, mixed berries, honey.
   Instructions: Layer Greek yogurt with granola and mixed berries; sprinkle with honey for a pleasant and protein-rich parfait.

 2. Avocado Toast: Ingredients: Whole grain bread, ripe avocado, salt, pepper, red pepper flakes (optional).
   Instructions: Spread mashed avocado over toast, sprinkle with salt, pepper, and red pepper flakes if preferred for a filling snack.

3. Hummus and Veggie Sticks:
   Ingredients: Hummus, carrot sticks,
cucumber slices, bell pepper strips.
   Instructions: Dip vegetable sticks in
hummus for a crispy and
nutrient-packed snack.

4. Fruit and Nut Trail Mix: Ingredients:
Mixed nuts (almonds, walnuts,
cashews), dried fruits (apricots,
cranberries), dark chocolate chips.
Instructions: Combine nuts, dried
fruits, and chocolate chips for a
customized and energy-boosting trail
mix.

5. Cucumber and Cream Cheese Bites:
Ingredients: Cucumber slices, cream
cheese, dill.

Instructions: Spread cream cheese
over cucumber slices, sprinkle with dill
for a delicious and low-carb snack.

6. Energy Balls:

Ingredients: Rolled oats, nut butter,
honey, chia seeds, dark chocolate
chips.

Instructions: Mix ingredients, form
into balls, and chill for a fast and
healthy energy-boosting snack.

7. Rice Cake with Almond Butter and
Banana:

Ingredients: Rice cake, almond butter, banana slices.

Instructions: Spread almond butter over a rice cake, top with banana slices for a simple and tasty snack.

8. Roasted Chickpeas:

Ingredients: Canned chickpeas, olive oil, cumin, paprika, salt.

Instructions: Toss chickpeas with olive oil and seasonings; roast until crispy for a delicious and protein-packed snack.

9. Cheese with Whole Grain Crackers:

Ingredients: Cheese slices or cubes, whole grain crackers.

Instructions: Pair cheese with whole grain crackers for a balanced and delicious snack.

10. Apple Slices with Peanut Butter:
Ingredients: Apple slices, peanut butter.
Instructions: Spread peanut butter over apple slices for a delightful blend of sweetness and nutty taste.

Salad recipes

Salads:

1. Classic Caesar Salad: Ingredients: Romaine lettuce, croutons, parmesan cheese, Caesar dressing.

Instructions: Toss lettuce with croutons, parmesan, and Caesar dressing for a classic salad.

2. Caprese Salad: Ingredients: Tomatoes, fresh mozzarella, basil, balsamic glaze.

Instructions: Arrange tomato and mozzarella slices with fresh basil; sprinkle with balsamic glaze.

3. Quinoa and Vegetable Salad: Ingredients: Quinoa, cherry tomatoes, cucumber, feta cheese, olive oil.

Instructions: Combine cooked quinoa with vegetables, feta, and olive oil for a healthful and delicious salad.

4. Spinach and Strawberry Salad: Ingredients: Baby spinach, strawberries, feta cheese, almonds, balsamic vinaigrette.
Instructions: Toss spinach with strawberries, feta, and almonds; sprinkle with balsamic vinaigrette.

5. Mango Avocado Salad: Ingredients: Mixed greens, mango, avocado, red onion, lime vinaigrette.
Instructions: Combine greens with mango, avocado, and red onion; garnish with lime vinaigrette.

Dessert recipes

1. Fresh Berry Parfait: Ingredients:
Mixed berries, Greek yogurt, granola,
honey.

Instructions: Layer fruit, yogurt, and
granola; sprinkle with honey for a
simple and healthful dessert.

2. Chocolate Avocado Mousse:
Ingredients: Avocado, chocolate
powder, honey, vanilla essence.

Instructions: Blend avocado, cocoa,
honey, and vanilla for a creamy and
decadent chocolate mousse.

3. Fruit Salad with Honey-Lime Drizzle:
   Ingredients: Assorted fruits (melon, berries, grapes), honey, lime juice.
   Instructions: Mix fruits; drizzle with honey and lime juice for a delightful fruit salad.

4. Baked Apple Crisp: Ingredients: Apples, oats, brown sugar, cinnamon, vanilla ice cream.
   Instructions: Bake sliced apples with a crumbly oat topping; serve warm with vanilla ice cream.

5. Chia Seed Pudding with Berries:a
   Ingredients: Chia seeds, almond milk, vanilla essence, assorted berries.

Instructions: Mix chia seeds, almond milk, and vanilla; chill until thickened, then top with berries.

6. Lemon Sorbet: Ingredients: Lemon juice, sugar, water.
Instructions: Make a simple syrup with sugar and water, combine with lemon juice, freeze, and churn for a pleasant sorbet.

7. Coconut Mango Rice Pudding: Ingredients: Arborio rice, coconut milk, mango, shredded coconut.
Instructions: Cook rice in coconut milk, toss in mango, then top with shredded coconut for a tropical rice pudding.

8. Peach Cobbler: Ingredients: Fresh peaches, flour, sugar, cinnamon, butter.

Instructions: Mix sliced peaches with a cinnamon-sugar mixture; top with a buttery crumble and bake for a traditional cobbler.

9. No-Bake Strawberry Cheesecake Cups:

Ingredients: Cream cheese, graham cracker crumbs, strawberries, whipped cream.

Instructions: Layer cream cheese mixture with graham cracker crumbs and strawberries; top with whipped cream for a simple and tasty dessert.

10. Dark Chocolate-Dipped Strawberries:

 Ingredients: Fresh strawberries, dark chocolate.

  Instructions: Melt dark chocolate, dip strawberries, and let them set for a beautiful and delightful dessert.

Chapter five

Nutrient-Rich Meals for Bone Health

Focusing on elements that improve bone strength and general wellness.

1. Salmon and Quinoa Bowl:
Salmon:Rich in omega-3 fatty acids and vitamin D, vital for bone health. Quinoa: High in magnesium, boosting calcium absorption for stronger bones. Leafy Greens Spinach or kale for extra calcium and vitamin K.

2. Mushroom with Spinach Omelette:
  Eggs: Good source of vitamin D,
necessary for calcium absorption.
  Mushrooms: Provide vitamin D when
exposed to sunshine; also include
copper for bone development.
  Spinach: High in calcium and vitamin
K.

3. Greek Yogurt Parfait with Nuts:
  Greek Yogurt:Packed with calcium
and protein.
  Berries:Rich in antioxidants and
vitamin C, boosting collagen formation
for bone development.
  Nuts (Almonds or Walnuts): Provide
calcium, magnesium, and healthy fats.

4. Spinach and Chickpea Salad:
   Spinach: High in calcium, vitamin K,
and magnesium.
   Chickpeas: Good source of protein,
calcium, and phosphorus.
   Olive Oil: Contains anti-inflammatory
ingredients for general wellness.

5. Sweet Potato and Black Bean Bowl:
   Sweet Potatoes:High in potassium and
vitamin C, helpful for bone density.
   Black Beans: Rich in magnesium,
calcium, and zinc.
Broccoli:Contains calcium, vitamin K,
and collagen-building elements.

6. Tofu Stir-Fry with Broccoli and
Brown Rice:
Tofu: Excellent plant-based source of
calcium and protein.
Broccoli: Rich in calcium, vitamin C,
and collagen-building elements.
Brown Rice:Provides magnesium and
phosphate for bone health.

7. Salad with Canned Sardines:
Sardines:High in calcium, vitamin D,
and omega-3 fatty acids.
Leafy Greens:Kale or arugula for extra
calcium and vitamin K.
Cherry Tomatoes:Contain antioxidants
boosting bone health.

8. Cottage Cheese and Pineapple Bowl:
Cottage Cheese:Good source of calcium
and protein.
Pineapple:Rich in manganese, helping
in bone growth and mineralization.

9. Lentil Soup with Kale:
Lentils:Provide protein, fiber, and
important minerals including
magnesium and phosphorus.
Kale:High in calcium, vitamin K, and
antioxidants.

10. Chicken and Vegetable Stir-Fry
with Whole Grain Rice:
Chicken:Good source of protein,
phosphorus, and vitamin D.

Vegetables (Broccoli, Bell Peppers):
Contain calcium, vitamin C, and other
bone-supporting elements.
Whole Grain Rice:Offers magnesium
and fiber.

Incorporating these nutrient-rich
foods into your diet delivers a balanced
combination of vitamins and minerals
important for bone health, including
calcium, vitamin D, magnesium, and
phosphorus. Remember to keep a
diverse and well-balanced diet for
general well-being.

Digestive Health Boosters

Recipes highlighting components that improve digestive well-being for elders.

1. Overnight Oats with Fiber and Berries:
Rolled Oats: High in soluble fiber for digestive regularity.
Chia Seeds:Provide extra fiber and omega-3 fatty acids.
Berries (Blueberries, Raspberries):Rich in antioxidants and fiber.

2. Probiotic-Rich Yogurt Parfait:
Greek Yogurt:Contains probiotics for a healthy gut microbiota.

Bananas:Provide prebiotics that encourage the development of healthy microorganisms.
Granola:Adds fiber for intestinal wellness.

3. Ginger and Turmeric Infused Smoothie: Bananas: Offer potassium and soluble fiber.

Ginger:Known for its anti–inflammatory qualities and assisting digestion.
Turmeric:Contains curcumin, which may aid with digestive disorders.

4. Quinoa Salad with
Digestive-Friendly Vegetables:
Quinoa:High in fiber and protein.
Cucumber: Hydrating and helps
digestion.
Mint Leaves:Known for relaxing the
digestive tract.

5. Baked Salmon with Lemon and Dill:
Salmon: Rich in omega-3 fatty acids for
anti-inflammatory benefits.
Lemon: Aids digestion and offers a
blast of flavor.
Dill:Known for its relaxing impact on
the digestive tract.

6. Mango and Papaya Smoothie:
Mango: Contains digestive enzymes like amylases.
Papaya:Rich in papain, an enzyme that assists digestion.
Yogurt: Adds probiotics for digestive health.

7.Fennel and Citrus Salad:
Fennel: Known for its digestive benefits and calming effects.
  Orange Segments: High in vitamin C and fiber.
  Arugula:Contains enzymes that help digestion.

8. Whole Grain Toast with Avocado:
Whole Grain Bread: Provides fiber for intestinal health.
Avocado: Rich in healthful fats and fiber.
  Tomato Slices: Adds freshness and a dose of vitamins.

9. Lentil and Vegetable Soup:
Lentils:High in fiber and protein.
  Carrots and Celery: Provide extra fiber and minerals.
  Cumin and Turmeric:Spices recognized for their digestive benefits.

10. Pineapple and Mint Infused Water:
Pineapple: Contains bromelain, an
enzyme helping digestion.

Mint Leaves:Known for relaxing the
digestive tract.

Cucumber Slices: Add freshness and
moisture.

Incorporating these meals into a
senior's diet may help to digestive
well-being by offering a combination of
fiber, probiotics, and
digestive-friendly components.
Additionally, keeping hydrated is vital
for having a healthy digestive tract.

Chapter six

Brain-Boosting Ingredients

Exploring foods recognized for cognitive advantages good for elderly

1. Blueberry and Walnut Smoothie:
Blueberries:Packed with antioxidants that may postpone brain aging.
Walnuts:High in omega-3 fatty acids for brain function.

2. Salmon and Avocado Salad:
Salmon: Rich in omega-3 fatty acids for cognitive function.
   Avocado:Contains monounsaturated fats and vitamin K for brain health.

3. Turmeric and Spinach Omelette:
Turmeric: Contains curcumin, which
has anti-inflammatory and antioxidant
effects.
  Spinach:High in folate and iron,
promoting cognitive development.

4. Whole Grain Porridge with Berries:
Whole Grains: Provide a continuous
supply of energy for the brain.
Berries (Strawberries,
Blueberries):Rich in antioxidants.

5. Broccoli and Cauliflower Stir-Fry:
Broccoli: High in choline, aiding brain
growth.

Cauliflower: Contains choline and antioxidants.

6. Dark Chocolate and Almond Snack:
Dark Chocolate:Contains flavonoids, caffeine, and antioxidants for cognitive function.
 Almonds:Rich in vitamin E, an antioxidant associated to brain health.

7. Eggplant and Tomato Bake:
Eggplant: Contains nasunin, an antioxidant that preserves brain cell membranes.
 Tomatoes: High in lycopene, which may protect against cognitive degeneration.

8. Green Tea with Lemon:
Green Tea: Contains caffeine and L-theanine, increasing alertness and attention.

  Lemon:Adds vitamin C, which may protect against cognitive deterioration.

9. Quinoa Salad with Kale and Pomegranate:
Quinoa: Provides complex carbs for sustained energy.

  Kale:High in vitamin K and antioxidants.

  Pomegranate Seeds:Contain polyphenols with possible cognitive advantages.

10. Cottage Cheese with Pineapple:
Cottage Cheese: A source of protein and
B-complex vitamins for brain health.
   Pineapple:Contains antioxidants and
vitamin C.

Incorporating these brain-boosting
items into a senior's diet may help to
cognitive well-being. A balanced and
diverse diet rich in nutrients,
antioxidants, and healthy fats
improves brain function and may help
avoid age-related cognitive decline.

Chapter seven

Adapting Elimination Diets to Age-Related Challenges

Tips for treating typical nutritional issues in the 40-60 age group.

Bone Health: Incorporate Calcium-Rich Foods: Include dairy products, fortified plant-based milk, leafy greens, and nuts to maintain bone health and minimize the risk of osteoporosis.

2. Joint Health: Omega-3 Fatty Acids:Include fatty seafood like salmon, walnuts, and flaxseeds to help decrease inflammation and improve joint health.
Turmeric and Ginger: Use these anti-inflammatory spices in cooking to possibly ease joint discomfort.

3. Heart Health: Heart-Healthy Fats:Choose sources of unsaturated fats, such as avocados, olive oil, and almonds, to promote cardiovascular health.
Fiber-Rich Foods: Include whole grains, fruits, and vegetables to help maintain healthy cholesterol levels.

4. Digestive Health: Probiotics:
Incorporate yogurt, kefir, and
fermented foods to boost gut health
and relieve digestive difficulties.
   Fiber Intake:Ensure an appropriate
intake of fiber from whole grains,
fruits, and vegetables for regular bowel
movements.

5. Metabolism and Weight
Management: Lean Proteins: Opt for
lean protein sources including chicken,
fish, tofu, and lentils to boost muscle
mass and metabolism.
Balanced Meals: Include a balance of
protein, healthy fats, and complex
carbs in each meal for sustained energy.

6. Cognitive Health: Antioxidant-Rich
Foods:Include berries, dark leafy
greens, and colorful veggies to boost
brain health and lower oxidative stress.
Omega-3 Fatty Acids:Consume fatty
fish or try omega-3 supplements for
cognitive function.

7. Blood Sugar Management: Whole
Grains: Choose whole grains over
processed carbs to help regulate blood
sugar levels.

Portion Control: Be cautious of portion
proportions to reduce blood sugar
spikes and crashes.

8. Eye Health: Vitamin A-Rich
Foods:Include carrots, sweet potatoes,
and leafy greens for eye health.
 Omega-3 Fatty Acids: Incorporate fish
or flaxseeds for possible advantages to
eye health.

9. Hydration: Water-Rich
Foods:Consume hydrating foods like
cucumbers, watermelon, and celery in
addition to drinking an appropriate
quantity of water everyday.

10. Flexibility and Adaptability:
Individualized Approach: Consider
personal preferences,

dietary limitations, and health concerns to personalize the elimination diet to individual requirements.

  Consultation with Healthcare Professionals:Seek help from healthcare specialists, especially a qualified dietitian, to build a specific and sustainable elimination diet plan.

Addressing age-related issues demands a comprehensive approach, addressing not just food modifications but also lifestyle aspects such as regular physical exercise and stress management. Always speak with healthcare specialists before making large changes to the diet, particularly for persons with specific health issues.

Managing Inflammation via Diet

1. Turmeric-Ginger Smoothie: Blend together pineapple, ginger, turmeric, Greek yogurt, and a touch of honey for a delicious anti-inflammatory smoothie.

2. fish and Quinoa Bowl: Grill fish and serve over a bed of quinoa, complemented with sautéed dark leafy greens and a sprinkle of olive oil.

3. Chia Seed Pudding with Berries: Mix chia seeds with almond milk, vanilla essence, and top with fresh berries for a healthful and anti-inflammatory dessert or snack.

4. Vegetarian Stir-Fry with Tofu:
Stir-fry colorful veggies and tofu with a
soy-ginger sauce, served over brown
rice for a simple and
inflammation-friendly dinner.

Quick and Easy Meals for Busy Seniors

1. Microwaveable Quinoa and Vegetable
Bowl: Combine pre-cooked quinoa,
mixed veggies, and a sprinkling of feta
cheese for a fast and healthy lunch.

2. Greek Yogurt Parfait with Granola:
Layer Greek yogurt with granola and
fresh fruit for a quick and tasty
breakfast or snack.

3. Whole Grain Wrap with Hummus
and vegetables: Spread hummus on a
whole grain wrap, add sliced
vegetables, and roll it up for a simple
and healthful lunch.

4. Rotisserie Chicken Salad: Shred
rotisserie chicken and combine with
mixed greens, cherry tomatoes, and a
basic vinaigrette for an
easy-to-assemble salad.

1. Grilled Vegetable Skewers: Bring a colorful dish of grilled vegetable skewers to offer at parties, giving a delightful and elimination-diet-friendly choice.

2. Fruit Salad with Mint-Lime Dressing: Create a delightful fruit salad with a mint-lime dressing for a lively and health-conscious addition to social occasions.

3. Chicken Lettuce Wraps: Prepare chicken lettuce wraps with a choice of toppings, giving a delightful and adaptable alternative for parties.

Seasonal Eating for Seniors

1. Summer Berry Salad: Combine fresh strawberries, blueberries, and raspberries with spinach, feta, and a balsamic vinaigrette for a seasonal and healthful salad.

2. Autumn Roasted veggies: Roast a combination of seasonal veggies including butternut squash, Brussels sprouts, and carrots with herbs for a tasty side dish.

3. Winter Citrus Salad: Create a citrus salad with segments of oranges and grapefruits, combined with arugula

and a zesty vinaigrette for a bright and seasonal alternative.

4. Spring Asparagus Stir-Fry: Stir-fry fresh asparagus, snap peas, and other spring veggies with tofu or lean protein for a light and seasonal supper.

These recipes and advice cater to varied nutritional demands, giving delectable and simple alternatives for seniors controlling inflammation, living busy lives, navigating social gatherings, and appreciating seasonal eating. Always speak with healthcare specialists for specific recommendations based on unique health situations.

chapter eight

Tips for Successful Long-Term Dietary Changes

Practical tips on keeping a healthy diet as a long-term lifestyle

1. Start Gradually: Implement adjustments gently to allow for acclimation and improved adherence to the new food habits.

2. Set Realistic objectives: Define feasible and realistic objectives, considering personal preferences, lifestyle, and health circumstances.

3. Diversify Your Diet: Embrace a range of foods to guarantee a well-rounded and nutritionally balanced diet, making it more fun and sustainable.

4. Meal Planning: Plan meals ahead to minimize last-minute bad choices and guarantee a balanced intake of nutrients.

5. Include Favorites in Moderation: Allow for occasional indulgences or favorite meals to retain pleasure while remaining cautious of portion proportions.

6. Hydration is Key: Stay appropriately hydrated by adding water, herbal teas, and hydrating meals into your daily routine.

7. Listen to Your Body: Pay attention to hunger and fullness signals, developing a balanced relationship with food.

8. Experiment with Cooking: Try various recipes and cooking techniques to find entertaining and healthful ways to make meals.

9. Seek Support: Share your nutritional objectives with friends, family, or a support group to obtain encouragement and accountability.

10. Incorporate Physical exercise: Combine a balanced diet with regular physical exercise for general well-being and better commitment to lifestyle changes.

11. Mindful Eating Practices: Practice mindful eating by enjoying each mouthful, identifying hunger and fullness, and appreciating the sensory experience of food.

12. Stay educated: Stay current on dietary knowledge and research to make educated decisions that correspond with your long-term health objectives.

13. Celebrate Progress: Acknowledge and celebrate victories along the road, acknowledging the good effect of consistent dietary modifications.

14. Adapt to Changes: Be open to modifying dietary habits as required, considering changes in health, lifestyle, or tastes over time.

15. Professional Guidance: Consult with healthcare specialists, such as dietitians or nutritionists, for specific guidance and assistance.

16. Keep a Food Journal: Maintain a food journal to monitor eating habits, detect trends, and increase self-awareness.

17. Stay Positive: Approach dietary changes with a positive perspective, focusing on the advantages and increases in general well-being.

18. Educate Yourself: Continuously educate yourself about nutrition, dietary choices, and their influence on health for long-term success.

Remember that effective long-term dietary adjustments are about developing a sustainable and happy lifestyle. Finding a balance that works for you and adjusting to your developing requirements is crucial to sustaining a balanced diet over time.

www.ingramcontent.com/pod-product-compliance
Lightning Source LLC
Chambersburg PA
CBHW060951260726
48661CB00005B/1832